The Easy Slow Cooker Cookbook

Must-Have Recipes for Beginners

By Mina Yu

Sommario

Introduction 5

Slow Cooker Breakfast Recipes 7

Introduction

We understand you are always seeking simpler methods to prepare your dishes. We additionally recognize you are possibly tired investing long hours in the kitchen cooking with many pans and pots.

Well, currently your search mores than! We located the perfect cooking area tool you can utilize from now on! We are discussing the Slow stove! These fantastic pots enable you to cook some of the most effective recipes ever before with minimum effort Slow cookers prepare your meals much easier as well as a lot much healthier! You do not require to be an expert in the kitchen area to prepare a few of one of the most scrumptious, flavorful, distinctive as well as abundant dishes!

All you need is your Slow cooker as well as the best ingredients! It will certainly show you that you can make some fantastic breakfasts, lunch meals, side recipes, poultry, meat and also fish dishes.

Ultimately yet notably, this cookbook supplies you some simple as well as pleasant desserts.

Slow Cooker Breakfast Recipes

Pork and Cranberries

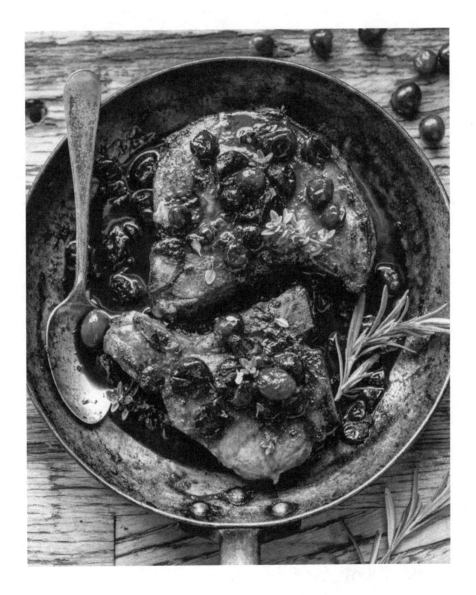

Preparation time: 10 minutes

Cooking time: 8 hours

Servings: 2

Ingredients:

- 1 pound pork tenderloin, roughly cubed

- ½ cup cranberries

- ½ cup red wine

- ½ teaspoon sweet paprika

- ½ teaspoon chili powder

- 1 tablespoon maple syrup

Directions:

1. In your slow cooker, mix the pork with the cranberries, wine and the other ingredients, toss, put the lid on and cook on Low for 8 hours.

2. Divide between plates and serve.

Nutrition: calories 400, fat 12, fiber 8, carbs 18, protein 20

Beef Chili

Preparation time: 10 minutes

Cooking time: 6 hours

Servings: 8

Ingredients:

- 3 chipotle chili peppers in adobo sauce, chopped

- 2 pounds beef steak, cubed

- 1 yellow onion, chopped

- 2 garlic cloves, minced

- 1 tablespoon chili powder

- Salt and black pepper to the taste

- 45 canned tomato puree

- ½ teaspoon cumin, ground

- 14 ounces beef stock

- 2 tablespoons cilantro, chopped

Directions:

1. In your Slow cooker, chipotle chilies with beef, onion, garlic, chili powder, salt, pepper, tomato puree, cumin and stock, stir, cover and cook on Low for 6 hours.

2. Add cilantro, stir, divide into bowls and serve for lunch.

Nutrition: calories 230, fat 8, fiber 2, carbs 12, protein 25

Pork Roast and Olives

Preparation time: 10 minutes

Cooking time: 6 hours

Servings: 2

Ingredients:

- 1 pound pork roast, sliced

- ½ cup black olives, pitted and halved

- ½ cup kalamata olives, pitted and halved

- 2 medium carrots, chopped

- ½ cup tomato sauce

- 1 small yellow onion, chopped

- 2 garlic cloves, minced

- 1 bay leaf

- Salt and black pepper to the taste

Directions:

1. In your slow cooker, mix the pork roast with the olives and the other ingredients, toss, put the lid on and cook on High for 6 hours.

2. Divide everything between plates and serve.

Nutrition: calories 360, fat 4, fiber 3, carbs 17, protein 27

Moist Pork Loin

Preparation time: 10 minutes

Cooking time: 5 hours

Servings: 8

Ingredients:

- 3 pound pork loin roast

- 1 teaspoon onion powder

- 1 teaspoon mustard powder

- 2 cups chicken stock

- 2 tablespoons olive oil

- ¼ cup cornstarch

- ¼ cup water

Directions:

1. In your Slow cooker, mix pork with onion powder, mustard powder, stock and oil, cover and cook on Low for 5 hours.

2. Transfer roast to a cutting board, slice and divide between plates.

3. Transfer cooking juices to a pan and heat it up over medium heat.

4. Add water and cornstarch, stir, cook until it thickens, drizzle over roast and serve for lunch.

Nutrition: calories 300, fat 11, fiber 1, carbs 10, protein 34

Beef Stew

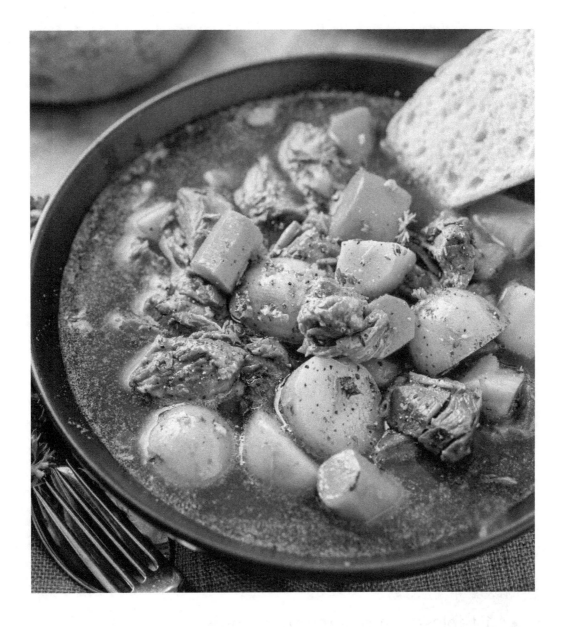

Preparation time: 10 minutes

Cooking time: 6 hours and 10 minutes

Servings: 2

Ingredients:

- 1 tablespoon olive oil

- 1 red onion, chopped

- 1 carrot, peeled and sliced

- 1 pound beef meat, cubed

- ½ cup beef stock

- ½ cup canned tomatoes, chopped

- 2 tablespoons tomato sauce

- 2 tablespoons balsamic vinegar

- 2 garlic cloves, minced

- ½ cup black olives, pitted and sliced

- 1 tablespoon rosemary, chopped

- Salt and black pepper to the taste

Directions:

1. Heat up a pan with the oil over medium-high heat, add the meat, brown for 10 minutes and transfer to your slow cooker.

2. Add the rest of the ingredients, toss, put the lid on and cook on High for 6 hours.

3. Divide between plates and serve right away!

Nutrition: calories 370, fat 14, fiber 6, carbs 26, protein 38

Lunch Meatloaf

Preparation time: 10 minutes

Cooking time: 4 hours

Servings: 8

Ingredients:

- ½ cup breadcrumbs

- 1 yellow onion, chopped

- 1 green bell pepper, chopped

- 2 eggs, whisked

- 2 tablespoons brown mustard

- ½ cup chili sauce

- Salt and black pepper to the taste

- 4 garlic cloves, minced

- ¼ teaspoon oregano, dried

- 2 pounds beef meat, ground

- ¼ teaspoon basil, dried

- Cooking spray

Directions:

1. In a bowl, mix beef with onion, breadcrumbs, bell pepper, mustard, chili sauce, eggs, salt, pepper, garlic, oregano and basil and stir well.

2. Line your Slow cooker with tin foil, grease with cooking spray, add beef meat, shape your meatloaf with your hands, cover and cook on Low for 4 hours.

3. Divide between plates and serve for lunch.

Nutrition: calories 253, fat 11, fiber 1, carbs 12, protein 25

Beef and Celery Stew

Preparation time: 10 minutes

Cooking time: 8 hours

Servings: 2

Ingredients:

- ½ cup beef stock

- 1 pound beef stew meat, cubed

- 1 cup celery, cubed

- ½ cup tomato sauce

- 2 carrots, chopped

- ½ cup mushrooms, halved

- ½ red onion, roughly chopped

- ½ tablespoon olive oil

- Salt and black pepper to the taste

- ¼ cup red wine

- 1 tablespoon parsley, chopped

Directions:

1. In your slow cooker, mix the beef with the stock, celery and the other ingredients, toss, put the lid on and cook on Low for 8 hours.

2. Divide the stew into bowls and serve.

Nutrition: calories 433, fat 20, fiber 4, carbs 14, protein 39

Mexican Lunch Mix

Preparation time: 10 minutes

Cooking time: 7 hours

Servings: 12

Ingredients:

- 12 ounces beer

- ¼ cup flour

- 2 tablespoons tomato paste

- 1 jalapeno pepper, chopped

- 1 bay leaf

- 4 teaspoons Worcestershire sauce

- 2 teaspoons red pepper flakes, crushed

- 1 and ½ teaspoons cumin, ground

- 2 teaspoons chili powder

- Salt and black pepper to the taste

- 2 garlic cloves, minced

- ½ teaspoon sweet paprika

- ½ teaspoon red vinegar

- 3 pounds pork shoulder butter, cubed

- 2 potatoes, chopped

- 1 yellow onion, chopped

Directions:

1. In your Slow cooker, mix pork with potatoes, onion, beef, flour, tomato paste, jalapeno, bay leaf, Worcestershire sauce, pepper flakes, cumin, chili powder, garlic, paprika and vinegar, toss, cover and cook on Low for 7 hours.

2. Divide between plates and serve for lunch.

Nutrition: calories 261, fat 12, fiber 2, carbs 16, protein 21

Tomato Pasta Mix

Preparation time: 10 minutes

Cooking time: 6 hours

Servings: 2

Ingredients:

- ½ pound beef stew meat, ground

- 1 red onion, chopped

- ½ teaspoon sweet paprika

- ½ teaspoon chili powder

- Salt and black pepper to the taste

- ½ teaspoon basil, dried

- ½ teaspoon parsley, dried

- 14 ounces canned tomatoes, chopped

- 1 cup chicken stock

- 1 cup short pasta

Directions:

1. In your slow cooker, mix the beef with the onion, paprika and the other ingredients except the pasta, toss, put the lid on and cook on Low for 5 hours and 30 minutes.

2. Add the pasta, stir, put the lid on again and cook on Low for 30 minutes more.

3. Divide everything between plates and serve.

Nutrition: calories 300, fat 6, fiber 8, carbs 18, protein 17

Sweet Turkey

Preparation time: 8 hours

Cooking time: 3 hours and 30 minutes

Servings: 12

Ingredients:

- 14 ounces chicken stock

- ¼ cup brown sugar

- ½ cup lemon juice

- ¼ cup lime juice

- ¼ cup sage, chopped

- ¼ cup cider vinegar

- 2 tablespoons mustard

- ¼ cup olive oil

- 1 tablespoon marjoram, chopped

- 1 teaspoon sweet paprika

- Salt and black pepper to the taste

- 1 teaspoon garlic powder

- 2 turkey breast halves, boneless and skinless

Directions:

1. In your blender, mix stock with brown sugar, lemon juice, lime juice, sage, vinegar, mustard, oil, marjoram, paprika, salt, pepper and garlic powder and pulse well.

2. Put turkey breast halves in a bowl, add blender mix, cover and leave aside in the fridge for 8 hours.

3. Transfer everything to your Slow cooker, cover and cook on High for 3 hours and 30 minutes.

4. Divide between plates and serve for lunch.

Nutrition: calories 219, fat 4, fiber 1, carbs 5, protein 36

Honey Lamb Roast

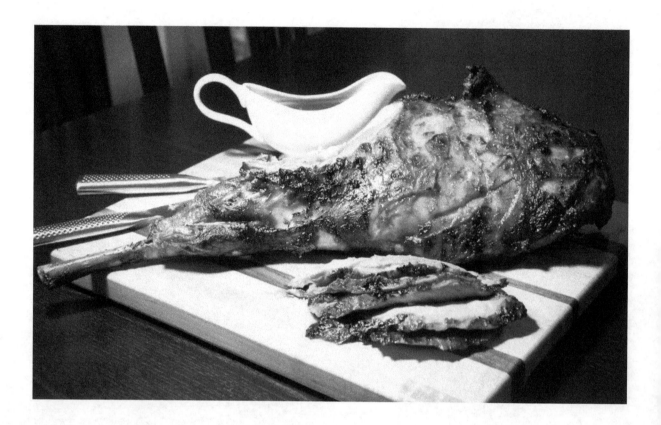

Preparation time: 10 minutes

Cooking time: 7 hours

Servings: 2

Ingredients:

- 1 pound lamb roast, sliced

- 3 tablespoons honey

- ½ tablespoon basil, dried

- ½ tablespoons oregano, dried

- 1 tablespoon garlic, minced

- 1 tablespoon olive oil

- Salt and black pepper to the taste

- ½ cup beef stock

Directions:

1. In your slow cooker, mix the lamb roast with the honey, basil and the other ingredients, toss well, put the lid on and cook on Low for 7 hours.

2. Divide everything between plates and serve.

Nutrition: calories 374, fat 6, fiber 8, carbs 29, protein 6

Beef Strips

Preparation time: 10 minutes

Cooking time: 6 hours

Servings: 4

Ingredients:

- ½ pound baby mushrooms, sliced

- 1 yellow onion, chopped

- 1 pound beef sirloin steak, cubed

- Salt and black pepper to the taste

- 1/3 cup red wine

- 2 teaspoons olive oil

- 2 cups beef stock

- 1 tablespoon Worcestershire sauce

Directions:

1. In your Slow cooker, mix beef strips with onion, mushrooms, salt, pepper, wine, olive oil, beef stock and Worcestershire sauce, toss, cover and cook on Low for 6 hours.

2. Divide between plates and serve for lunch.

Nutrition: calories 212, fat 7, fiber 1, carbs 8, protein 26

Worcestershire Beef Mix

Preparation time: 10 minutes

Cooking time: 8 hours

Servings: 2

Ingredients:

- 1 pound beef stew meat, cubed

- 1 teaspoon chili powder

- Salt and black pepper to the taste

- 1 cup beef stock

- 1 and ½ tablespoons Worcestershire sauce

- 1 teaspoon garlic, minced

- 2 ounces cream cheese, soft

- Cooking spray

Directions:

1. Grease your slow cooker with the cooking spray, and mix the beef with the stock and the other ingredients inside.

2. Put the lid on, cook on Low for 8 hours, divide between plates and serve.

Nutrition: calories 372, fat 6, fiber 9, carbs 18, protein 22

BBQ Chicken Thighs

Preparation time: 10 minutes

Cooking time: 5 hours

Servings: 6

Ingredients:

- 6 chicken thighs, skinless and boneless

- 1 yellow onion, chopped

- ½ teaspoon poultry seasoning

- 14 ounces canned tomatoes, chopped

- 8 ounces tomato sauce

- ½ cup bbq sauce

- 1 teaspoon garlic powder

- ¼ cup orange juice

- ½ teaspoon hot pepper sauce

- ¾ teaspoon oregano, dried

- Salt and black pepper to the taste

Directions:

1. In your Slow cooker, mix chicken with onion, poultry seasoning, tomatoes, tomato sauce, bbq sauce, garlic powder, orange juice, pepper sauce, oregano, salt and pepper, toss, cover and cook on Low for 5 hours.

2. Divide between plates and serve with the sauce drizzled on top.

Nutrition: calories 211, fat 9, fiber 2, carbs 12, protein 23

Chickpeas Stew

Preparation time: 10 minutes

Cooking time: 6 hours

Servings: 2

Ingredients:

- ½ tablespoon olive oil

- 1 red onion, chopped

- 2 garlic cloves, minced

- 1 red chili pepper, chopped

- ¼ cup carrots, chopped

- 6 ounces canned tomatoes, chopped

- 6 ounces canned chickpeas, drained

- ½ cup chicken stock

- 1 bay leaf

- ½ teaspoon coriander, ground

- A pinch of red pepper flakes

- ½ tablespoon parsley, chopped

- Salt and black pepper to the taste

Directions:

1. In your slow cooker, mix the chickpeas with the onion, garlic and the other ingredients, toss, put the lid on and cook on Low for 6 hours.

2. Divide into bowls and serve.

Nutrition: calories 462, fat 7, fiber 9, carbs 30, protein 17

Fall Slow Cooker Roast

Preparation time: 10 minutes

Cooking time: 6 hours

Servings: 6

Ingredients:

- 2 sweet potatoes, cubed

- 2 carrots, chopped

- 2 pounds beef chuck roast, cubed

- ¼ cup celery, chopped

- 1 tablespoon canola oil

- 2 garlic cloves, minced

- 1 yellow onion, chopped

- 1 tablespoon flour

- 1 tablespoon brown sugar

- 1 tablespoon sugar

- 1 teaspoon cumin, ground

- Salt and black pepper to the taste

- ¾ teaspoon coriander, ground

- ½ teaspoon oregano, dried

- 1 teaspoon chili powder

- 1/8 teaspoon cinnamon powder

- ¾ teaspoon orange peel grated

- 15 ounces tomato sauce

Directions:

1. In your Slow cooker, mix potatoes with carrots, beef cubes, celery, oil, garlic, onion, flour, brown sugar, sugar, cumin, salt pepper, coriander, oregano, chili powder, cinnamon, orange peel and tomato sauce, stir, cover and cook on Low for 6 hours.

2. Divide into bowls and serve for lunch.

Nutrition: calories 278, fat 12, fiber 2, carbs 16, protein 25

Lentils Soup

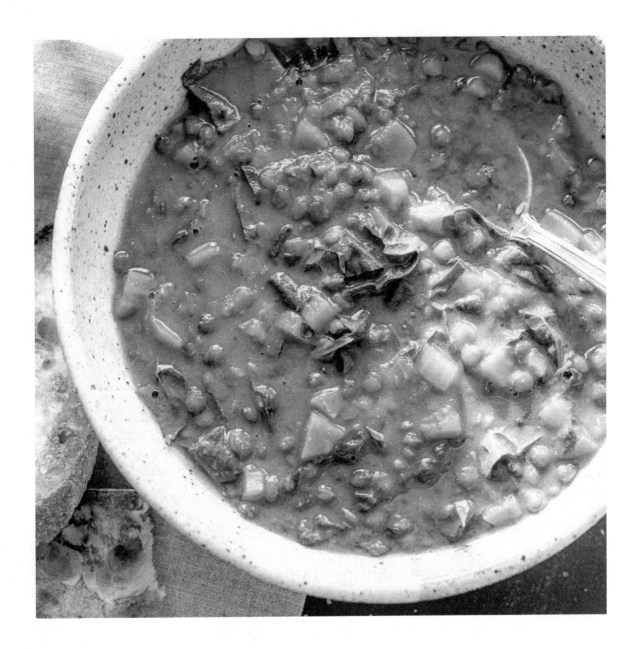

Preparation time: 10 minutes

Cooking time: 4 hours

Servings: 2

Ingredients:

- 2 garlic cloves, minced

- 1 carrot, chopped

- 1 red onion, chopped

- 3 cups veggie stock

- 1 cup brown lentils

- ½ teaspoon cumin, ground

- 1 bay leaf

- 1 tablespoon lime juice

- 1 tablespoon cilantro, chopped

- Salt and black pepper to the taste

Directions:

1. In your slow cooker, mix the lentils with the garlic, carrot and the other ingredients, toss, put the lid on and cook on High for 4 hours.

2. Ladle the soup into bowls and serve.

Nutrition: calories 361, fat 7, fiber 7, carbs 16, protein 5

Creamy Chicken

Preparation time: 10 minutes

Cooking time: 8 hours and 30 minutes

Servings: 6

Ingredients:

- 10 ounces canned cream of chicken soup

- Salt and black pepper to the taste

- A pinch of cayenne pepper

- 3 tablespoons flour

- 1 pound chicken breasts, skinless, boneless and cubed

- 1 celery rib, chopped

- ½ cup green bell pepper, chopped

- ¼ cup yellow onion, chopped

- 10 ounces peas

- 2 tablespoons pimientos, chopped

Directions:

1. In your Slow cooker, mix cream of chicken with salt, pepper, cayenne and flour and whisk well.

2. Add chicken, celery, bell pepper and onion, toss, cover and cook on Low for 8 hours.

3. Add peas and pimientos, stir, cover and cook on Low for 30 minutes more.

4. Divide into bowls and serve for lunch.

Nutrition: calories 200, fat 3, fiber 4, carbs 16, protein 17

Chicken Soup

Preparation time: 10 minutes

Cooking time: 7 hours

Servings: 2

Ingredients:

- ½ pound chicken breast, skinless, boneless and cubed

- 3 cups chicken stock

- 1 red onion, chopped

- 1 garlic clove, minced

- ½ celery stalk, chopped

- ¼ teaspoon chili powder

- ¼ teaspoon sweet paprika

- A pinch of salt and black pepper

- A pinch of cayenne pepper

- 1 tablespoon lemon juice

- ½ tablespoon chives, chopped

Directions:

1. In your slow cooker, mix the chicken with the stock, onion and the other ingredients, toss, put the lid on and cook on Low for 7 hours.

2. Divide into bowls and serve right away.

Nutrition: calories 351, fat 6, fiber 7, carbs 17, protein 16

Chicken Stew

Preparation time: 10 minutes

Cooking time: 8 hours

Servings: 6

Ingredients:

- 32 ounces chicken stock

- 3 spicy chicken sausage links, cooked and sliced

- 28 ounces canned tomatoes, chopped

- 1 yellow onion, chopped

- 1 cup lentils

- 1 carrot, chopped

- 2 garlic cloves, minced

- 1 celery rib, chopped

- ½ teaspoon thyme, dried

- Salt and black pepper to the taste

Directions:

1. In your Slow cooker, mix stock with sausage, tomatoes, onion, lentils, carrot, garlic, celery, thyme, salt and pepper, stir, cover and cook on Low for 8 hours.

2. Divide into bowls and serve for lunch.

Nutrition: calories 231, fat 4, fiber 12, carbs 31, protein 15

Lime and Thyme Chicken

Preparation time: 10 minutes

Cooking time: 6 hours

Servings: 2

Ingredients:

- 1 pound chicken thighs, boneless and skinless

- Juice of 1 lime

- 1 tablespoon lime zest, grated

- 2 teaspoons olive oil

- ½ cup tomato sauce

- 2 garlic cloves, minced

- 1 tablespoon thyme, chopped

- Salt and black pepper to the taste

Directions:

1. In your slow cooker, mix the chicken with the lime juice, zest and the other ingredients, toss, put the lid on and cook on High for 6 hours.

2. Divide between plates and serve right away.

Nutrition: calories 324, fat 7, fiber 8, carbs 20, protein 17

Lemon Chicken

Preparation time: 10 minutes

Cooking time: 5 hours

Servings: 6

Ingredients:

- 6 chicken breast halves, skinless and bone in

- Salt and black pepper to the taste

- 1 teaspoon oregano, dried

- ¼ cup water

- 2 tablespoons butter

- 3 tablespoons lemon juice

- 2 garlic cloves, minced

- 1 teaspoon chicken bouillon granules

- 2 teaspoons parsley, chopped

Directions:

1. In your Slow cooker, mix chicken with salt, pepper, water, butter, lemon juice, garlic and chicken granules, stir, cover and cook on Low for 5 hours.

2. Add parsley, stir, divide between plates and serve for lunch.

Nutrition: calories 336, fat 10, fiber 1, carbs 1, protein 46

Shrimp Gumbo

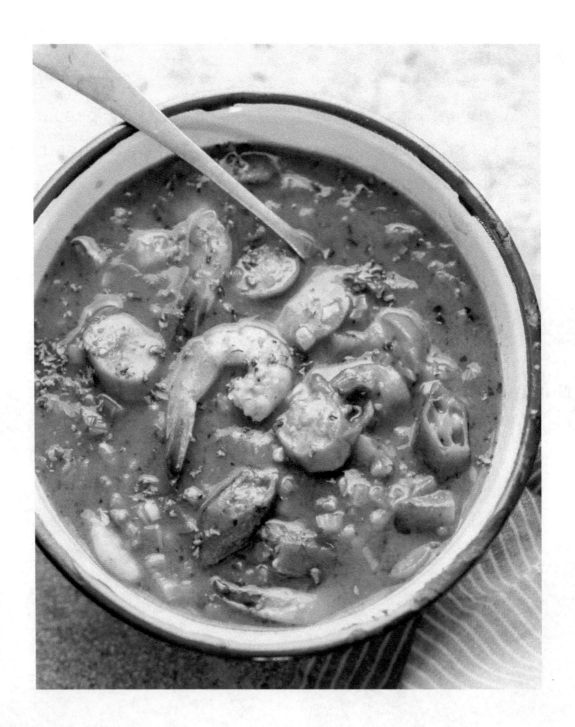

Preparation time: 10 minutes

Cooking time: 2 hours

Servings: 2

Ingredients:

- 1 pound shrimp, peeled and deveined

- ½ pound pork sausage, sliced

- 1 red onion, chopped

- ½ green bell pepper, chopped

- 1 red chili pepper, minced

- ½ teaspoon cumin, ground

- ½ teaspoon coriander, ground

- Salt and black pepper to the taste

- 1 cup tomato sauce

- ½ cup chicken stock

- ½ tablespoon Cajun seasoning

- ½ teaspoon oregano, dried

Directions:

1. In your slow cooker, mix the shrimp with the sausage, onion and the other ingredients, toss, put the lid on and cook on High for 2 hours.

2. Divide into bowls and serve.

Nutrition: calories 721, fat 36.7, fiber 3.7, carbs 18.2, protein 76.6

Pesto Pork Shanks

Preparation time: 10 minutes

Cooking time: 7 hours

Servings: 2

Ingredients:

- 1 and ½ pounds pork shanks

- 1 tablespoon olive oil

- 2 tablespoons basil pesto

- 1 red onion, sliced

- 1 cup beef stock

- ½ cup tomato paste

- 4 garlic cloves, minced

- 1 tablespoon oregano, chopped

- Zest and juice of 1 lemon

- A pinch of salt and black pepper

Directions:

1. In your slow cooker, mix the pork shanks with the oil, pesto and the other ingredients, toss, put the lid on and cook on Low for 7 hours.

2. Divide everything between plates and serve for lunch.

Nutrition: calories 372, fat 7, fiber 5, carbs 12, protein 37

Chicken Thighs Mix

Preparation time: 10 minutes

Cooking time: 6 hours

Servings: 6

Ingredients:

- 2 and ½ pounds chicken thighs, skinless and boneless

- 1 and ½ tablespoon olive oil

- 2 yellow onions, chopped

- 1 teaspoon cinnamon powder

- ¼ teaspoon cloves, ground

- ¼ teaspoon allspice, ground

- Salt and black pepper to the taste

- A pinch of saffron

- A handful pine nuts

- A handful mint, chopped

Directions:

1. In a bowl, mix oil with onions, cinnamon, allspice, cloves, salt, pepper and saffron, whisk and transfer to your slow cooker.

2. Add the chicken, toss well, cover and cook on Low for 6 hours.

3. Sprinkle pine nuts and mint on top before serving,

Nutrition: calories 223, fat 3, fiber 2, carbs 6, protein 13

Potato Stew

Preparation time: 10 minutes

Cooking time: 5 hours and 5 minutes

Servings: 4

Ingredients:

- ½ tablespoon olive oil

- 1 pound gold potatoes, peeled and cut into wedges

- 1 red onion, sliced

- 1 cup tomato paste

- ½ cup beef stock

- 1 carrot, sliced

- 1 red bell pepper, cubed

- 4 garlic cloves, minced

- 1 teaspoon sweet paprika

- 1 tablespoon chives, chopped

Directions:

1. Heat up a pan with the oil over medium-high heat, add the onion and garlic, sauté for 5 minutes and transfer to the slow cooker.

2. Add the potatoes and the other ingredients, toss, put the lid on and cook on Low for 5 hours.

3. Divide the stew into bowls and serve for lunch.

Nutrition: calories 273, fat 6, fiber 7, carbs 10, protein 17

Chicken and Stew

Preparation time: 10 minutes

Cooking time: 5 hours

Servings: 4

Ingredients:

- 4 chicken breasts, skinless and boneless

- 6 Italian sausages, sliced

- 5 garlic cloves, minced

- 1 white onion, chopped

- 1 teaspoon Italian seasoning

- A drizzle of olive oil

- 1 teaspoon garlic powder

- 29 ounces canned tomatoes, chopped

- 15 ounces tomato sauce

- 1 cup water

- ½ cup balsamic vinegar

Directions:

1. Put chicken and sausage slices in your slow cooker, add garlic, onion, Italian seasoning, oil, tomatoes, tomato sauce, garlic powder, water and the vinegar, cover and cook on High for 5 hours.

2. Stir the stew, divide between plates and serve for lunch

Nutrition: calories 267, fat 4, fiber 3, carbs 15, protein 13

Chicken and Rice

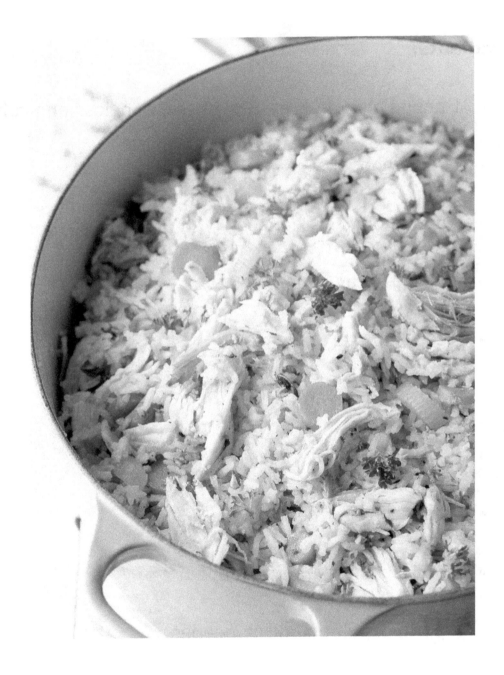

Preparation time: 10 minutes

Cooking time: 6 hours

Servings: 2

Ingredients:

- 1 pound chicken breast, skinless, boneless and cubed

- 1 red onion, sliced

- 2 spring onions, chopped

- Cooking spray

- 1 cup wild rice

- 2 cups chicken stock

- ½ teaspoon garam masala

- ½ teaspoon turmeric powder

- 1 tablespoon cilantro, chopped

- A pinch of salt and black pepper

Directions:

1. Grease the slow cooker with the cooking spray, add the chicken, rice, onion and the other ingredients, toss, put the lid on and cook on Low for 6 hours.

2. Divide the mix into bowls and serve for lunch.

Nutrition: calories 362, fat 8, fiber 8, carbs 10, protein 26

Chicken and Cabbage Mix

Preparation time: 10 minutes

Cooking time: 5 hours and 20 minutes

Servings: 6

Ingredients:

- 6 garlic cloves, minced

- 4 scallions, sliced

- 1 cup veggie stock

- 1 tablespoon olive oil

- 2 teaspoons sugar

- 1 tablespoon soy sauce

- 1 teaspoon ginger, minced

- 2 pounds chicken thighs, skinless and boneless

- 2 cups cabbage, shredded

Directions:

1. In your Slow cooker, mix stock with oil, scallions, garlic, sugar, soy sauce, ginger and chicken, stir, cover and cook on Low for 5 hours.

2. Transfer chicken to plates, add cabbage to the slow cooker, cover, cook on High for 20 minutes more, add next to the chicken and serve for lunch.

Nutrition: calories 240, fat 3, fiber 4, carbs 14, protein 10

Salmon Stew

Preparation time: 10 minutes

Cooking time: 2 hours

Servings: 4

Ingredients:

- 1 pound salmon fillets, boneless and roughly cubed

- 1 cup chicken stock

- ½ cup tomato paste

- ½ red onion, sliced

- 1 carrot, sliced

- 1 sweet potato, peeled and cubed

- 1 tablespoon cilantro, chopped

- Cooking spray

- ½ cup mild salsa

- 2 garlic cloves, minced

- A pinch of salt and black pepper

Directions:

1. In your slow cooker, mix the fish with the stock, tomato paste, onion and the other ingredients, toss gently, put the lid on and cook on Low for 2 hours

2. Divide the mix into bowls and serve for lunch.

Nutrition: calories 292, fat 6, fiber 7, carbs 12, protein 22

Pork and Chorizo Lunch Mix

Preparation time: 10 minutes

Cooking time: 4 hours

Servings: 8

Ingredients:

- 1 pound chorizo, ground

- 1 pound pork, ground

- 3 tablespoons olive oil

- 1 tomato, chopped

- 1 avocado, pitted, peeled and chopped

- Salt and black pepper to the taste

- 1 small red onion, chopped

- 2 tablespoons enchilada sauce

Directions:

1. Heat up a pan with the oil over medium-high heat, add pork, stir, brown for a couple of minutes, transfer to your slow cooker, add salt, pepper, chorizo, onion and enchilada sauce, stir, cover and cook on Low for 4 hours.

2. Divide between plates and serve with chopped tomato and avocado on top.

Nutrition: calories 300, fat 12, fiber 3, carbs 15, protein 17

Paprika Pork and Chickpeas

Preparation time: 10 minutes

Cooking time: 10 hours

Servings: 2

Ingredients:

- 1 red onion, sliced

- 1 pound pork stew meat, cubed

- 1 cup canned chickpeas, drained

- 1 cup beef stock

- 1 cup tomato paste

- ½ teaspoon sweet paprika

- ½ teaspoon turmeric powder

- A pinch of salt and black pepper

- 1 tablespoon hives, chopped

Directions:

1. In your slow cooker, mix the onion with the meat, chickpeas, stock and the other ingredients, toss, put the lid on and cook on Low for 10 hours.

2. Divide the mix between plates and serve for lunch.

Nutrition: calories 322, fat 6, fiber 6, carbs 9, protein 22

Lamb Stew

Preparation time: 10 minutes

Cooking time: 8 hours

Servings: 4

Ingredients:

- 1 and ½ pounds lamb meat, cubed

- ¼ cup flour

- Salt and black pepper to the taste

- 2 tablespoons olive oil

- 1 teaspoon rosemary, dried

- 1 onion, sliced

- ½ teaspoon thyme, dried

- 2 cups water

- 1 cup baby carrots

- 2 cups sweet potatoes, chopped

Directions:

1. In a bowl, mix lamb with flour and toss.

2. Heat up a pan with the oil over medium-high heat, add meat, brown it on all sides and transfer to your slow cooker.

3. Add onion, salt, pepper, rosemary, thyme, water, carrots and sweet potatoes, cover and cook on Low for 8 hours.

4. Divide lamb stew between plates and serve for lunch

Nutrition: calories 350, fat 8, fiber 3, carbs 20, protein 16

Beef and Cabbage

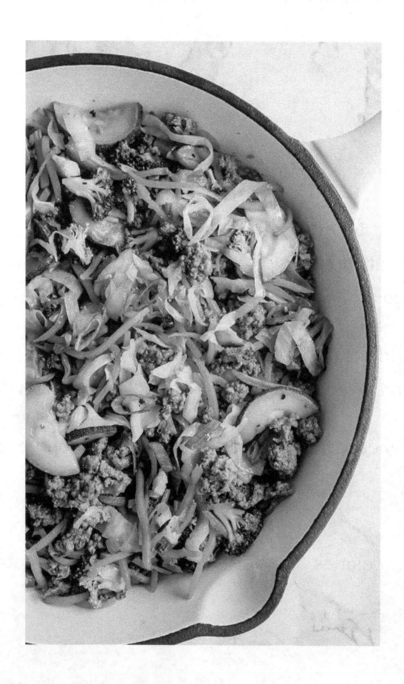

Preparation time: 10 minutes

Cooking time: 8 hours

Servings: 2

Ingredients:

- 1 pound beef stew meat, cubed

- 1 cup green cabbage, shredded

- 1 cup red cabbage, shredded

- 1 carrot, grated

- ½ cup water

- 1 cup tomato paste

- ½ teaspoon sweet paprika

- 1 tablespoon chives, chopped

- A pinch of salt and black pepper

Directions:

1. In your slow cooker, mix the beef with the cabbage, carrot and the other ingredients, toss, put the lid on and cook on Low for 8 hours.

2. Divide the mix between plates and serve for lunch.

Nutrition: calories 251, fat 6, fiber 7, carbs 12, protein 6

Lamb Curry

Preparation time: 10 minutes

Cooking time: 4 hours

Servings: 4

Ingredients:

- 1 and ½ tablespoons sweet paprika

- 3 tablespoons curry powder

- Salt and black pepper to the taste

- 2 pounds lamb meat, cubed

- 2 tablespoons olive oil

- 3 carrots, chopped

- 4 celery stalks, chopped

- 1 onion, chopped

- 4 celery stalks, chopped

- 1 cup chicken stock

- 4 garlic cloves minced

- 1 cup coconut milk

Directions:

1. Heat up a pan with the oil over medium-high heat, add lamb meat, brown it on all sides and transfer to your slow cooker.

2. Add stock, onions, celery and carrots to the slow cooker and stir everything gently.

3. In a bowl, mix paprika with a pinch of salt, black pepper and curry powder and stir.

4. Add spice mix to the cooker, also add coconut milk, cover, cook on High for 4 hours, divide into bowls and serve for lunch.

Nutrition: calories 300, fat 4, fiber 4, carbs 16, protein 13

Balsamic Beef Stew

Preparation time: 10 minutes

Cooking time: 6 hours

Servings: 2

Ingredients:

- 1 pound beef stew meat, cubed

- 1 teaspoon sweet paprika

- 1 red onion, sliced

- ½ cup mushrooms, sliced

- 1 carrot, peeled and cubed

- ½ cup tomatoes, cubed

- 1 tablespoon balsamic vinegar

- A pinch of salt and black pepper

- 1 teaspoon onion powder

- 1 teaspoon thyme, dried

- 1 cup beef stock

- 1 tablespoon cilantro, chopped

Directions:

1. In your slow cooker, mix the beef with the paprika, onion, mushrooms and the other ingredients except the cilantro, toss, put the lid on and cook on Low for 6 hours.

2. Divide into bowls and serve with the cilantro, sprinkled on top.

Nutrition: calories 322, fat 5, fiber 7, carbs 9, protein 16

Lamb and Bacon Stew

Preparation time: 10 minutes

Cooking time: 7 hours and 10 minutes

Servings: 6

Ingredients:

- 2 tablespoons flour

- 2 ounces bacon, cooked and crumbled

- 1 and ½ pounds lamb loin, chopped

- Salt and black pepper to the taste

- 1 garlic clove, minced

- 1 cup yellow onion, chopped

- 3 and ½ cups veggie stock

- 1 cup carrots, chopped

- 1 cup celery, chopped

- 2 cups sweet potatoes, chopped

- 1 tablespoon thyme, chopped

- 1 bay leaf

- 2 tablespoons olive oil

Directions:

1. Put lamb meat in a bowl, add flour, salt and pepper and toss to coat.

2. Heat up a pan with the oil over medium-high heat, add lamb, brown for 5 minutes on each side and transfer to your slow cooker.

3. Add onion, garlic, bacon, carrots, potatoes, bay leaf, stock, thyme and celery to the slow cooker as well, stir gently, cover and cook on Low for 7 hours.

4. Discard bay leaf, stir your stew, divide into bowls and serve for lunch

Nutrition: calories 360, fat 5, fiber 3, carbs 16, protein 17

Beef Curry

Preparation time: 10 minutes

Cooking time: 6 hours

Servings: 2

Ingredients:

- 1 pound beef stew meat

- 4 garlic cloves, minced

- 1 red onion, sliced

- 2 carrots, grated

- 1 tablespoon ginger, grated

- 2 tablespoons yellow curry paste

- 2 cups coconut milk

- A pinch of salt and black pepper

Directions:

1. In your slow cooker, mix the beef with the garlic, onion and the other ingredients, toss, put the lid on and cook on Low for 6 hours.

2. Divide the curry into bowls and serve for lunch.

Nutrition: calories 352, fat 6, fiber 7, carbs 9, protein 18

Sweet Potato Soup

Preparation time: 10 minutes

Cooking time: 5 hours and 20 minutes

Servings: 6

Ingredients:

- 5 cups veggie stock

- 3 sweet potatoes, peeled and chopped

- 2 celery stalks, chopped

- 1 cup yellow onion, chopped

- 1 cup milk

- 1 teaspoon tarragon, dried

- 2 garlic cloves, minced

- 2 cups baby spinach

- 8 tablespoons almonds, sliced

- Salt and black pepper to the taste

Directions:

1. In your slow cooker, mix stock with potatoes, celery, onion, milk, tarragon, garlic, salt and pepper, stir, cover and cook on High for 5 hours.

2. Blend soup using an immersion blender, add spinach and almonds, toss, cover and leave aside for 20 minutes.

3. Divide soup into bowls and serve for lunch.

Nutrition: calories 301, fat 5, fiber 4, carbs 12, protein 5

Chicken and Brussels Sprouts Mix

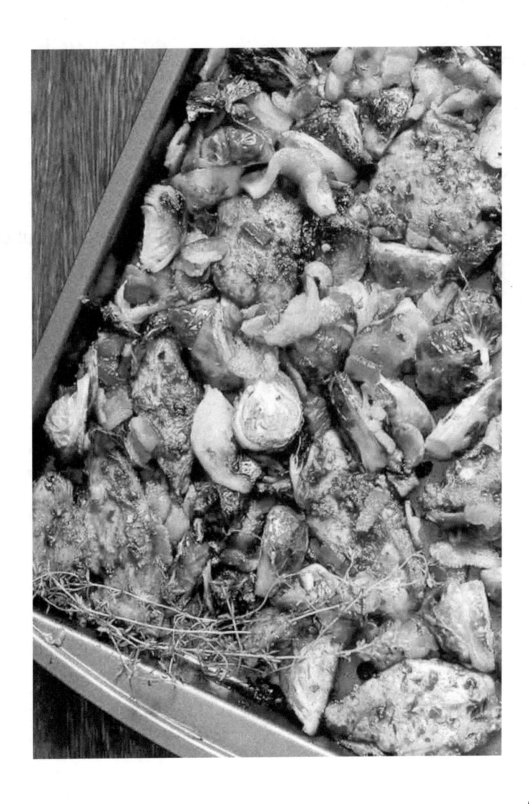

Preparation time: 10 minutes

Cooking time: 6 hours

Servings: 2

Ingredients:

- 1 pound chicken breast, skinless, boneless and cubed

- 1 red onion, sliced

- 1 cup Brussels sprouts, trimmed and halved

- 1 cup chicken stock

- ½ cup tomato paste

- A pinch of salt and black pepper

- 1 garlic clove, crushed

- 1 tablespoon thyme, chopped

- 1 tablespoon rosemary, chopped

Directions:

1. In your slow cooker, mix the chicken with the onion, sprouts and the other ingredients, toss, put the lid on and cook on Low for 6 hours.

2. Divide the mix between plates and serve for lunch.

Nutrition: calories 261, fat 7, fiber 6, carbs 8, protein 26

White Beans Stew

Preparation time: 10 minutes

Cooking time: 4 hours

Servings: 10

Ingredients:

- 2 pounds white beans

- 3 celery stalks, chopped

- 2 carrots, chopped

- 1 bay leaf

- 1 yellow onion, chopped

- 3 garlic cloves, minced

- 1 teaspoon rosemary, dried

- 1 teaspoon oregano, dried

- 1 teaspoon thyme, dried

- 10 cups water

- Salt and black pepper to the taste

- 28 ounces canned tomatoes, chopped

- 6 cups chard, chopped

Directions:

1. In your slow cooker, mix white beans with celery, carrots, bay leaf, onion, garlic, rosemary, oregano, thyme, water, salt, pepper, tomatoes and chard, cover and cook on High for 4 hours.

2. Stir, divide into bowls and serve for lunch,

Nutrition: calories 341, fat 8, fiber 12, carbs 20, protein 6

Chickpeas Stew

Preparation time: 10 minutes

Cooking time: 3 hours

Servings: 4

Ingredients:

- 2 cups canned chickpeas, drained and rinsed

- 1 cup tomato sauce

- ½ cup chicken stock

- 1 red onion, sliced

- 2 garlic cloves, minced

- 1 tablespoon thyme, chopped

- ½ teaspoon turmeric powder

- ½ teaspoon garam masala

- 2 carrots, chopped

- 3 celery stalks, chopped

- 2 tablespoons parsley, chopped

- A pinch of salt and black pepper

Directions:

1. In your slow cooker, mix the chickpeas with the tomato sauce, chicken stock and the other ingredients, toss, put the lid on and cook on High for 3 hours.

2. Divide into bowls and serve for lunch.

Nutrition: calories 300, fat 4, fiber 7, carbs 9, protein 22

Bulgur Chili

Preparation time: 10 minutes

Cooking time: 8 hours

Servings: 4

Ingredients:

- 2 cups white mushrooms, sliced

- ¾ cup bulgur, soaked in 1 cup hot water for 15 minutes and drained

- 2 cups yellow onion, chopped

- ½ cup red bell pepper, chopped

- 1 cup veggie stock

- 2 garlic cloves, minced

- 1 cup strong brewed coffee

- 14 ounces canned kidney beans, drained

- 14 ounces canned pinto beans, drained

- 2 tablespoons sugar

- 2 tablespoons chili powder

- 1 tablespoon cocoa powder

- 1 teaspoon oregano, dried

- 2 teaspoons cumin, ground

- 1 bay leaf

- Salt and black pepper to the taste

Directions:

1. In your Slow cooker, mix mushrooms with bulgur, onion, bell pepper, stock, garlic, coffee, kidney and pinto beans, sugar, chili powder, cocoa, oregano, cumin, bay leaf, salt and pepper, stir gently, cover and cook on Low for 12 hours.

2. Discard bay leaf, divide chili into bowls and serve for lunch.

Nutrition: calories 351, fat 4, fiber 6, carbs 20, protein 4

Eggplant Curry

Preparation time: 10 minutes

Cooking time: 3 hours

Servings: 2

Ingredients:

- 2 tablespoons olive oil

- 1 pound eggplant, cubed

- 2 tablespoons red curry paste

- 1 cup coconut milk

- ½ cup veggie stock

- 1 teaspoon turmeric powder

- ½ teaspoon rosemary, dried

- 4 kaffir lime leaves

Directions:

1. In your slow cooker, mix the eggplant with the oil, curry paste and the other ingredients, toss, put the lid on and cook on High for 3 hours.

2. Discard lime leaves, divide the curry into bowls and serve for lunch.

Nutrition: calories 281, fat 7, fiber 6, carbs 8, protein 22

Quinoa Chili

Preparation time: 10 minutes

Cooking time: 6 hours

Servings: 6

Ingredients:

- 2 cups veggie stock

- ½ cup quinoa

- 30 ounces canned black beans, drained

- 28 ounces canned tomatoes, chopped

- 1 green bell pepper, chopped

- 1 yellow onion, chopped

- 2 sweet potatoes, cubed

- 1 tablespoon chili powder

- 2 tablespoons cocoa powder

- 2 teaspoons cumin, ground

- Salt and black pepper to the taste

- ¼ teaspoon smoked paprika

Directions:

1. In your slow cooker, mix stock with quinoa, black beans, tomatoes, bell pepper, onion, sweet potatoes, chili powder, cocoa, cumin, paprika, salt and pepper, stir, cover and cook on High for 6 hours.

2. Divide into bowls and serve for lunch.

Nutrition: calories 342, fat 6, fiber 7, carbs 18, protein 4

Beef and Artichokes Stew

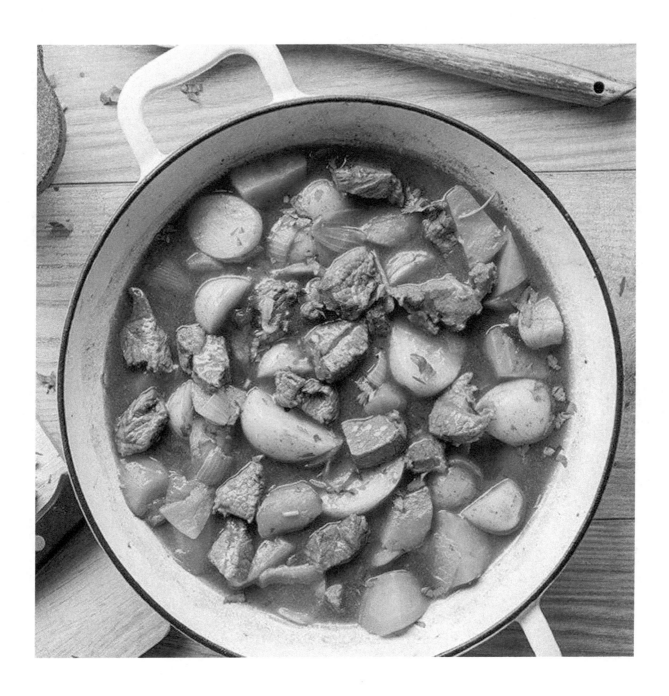

Preparation time: 10 minutes

Cooking time: 4 hours

Servings: 2

Ingredients:

- 1 pound beef stew meat, cubed

- 1 cup canned artichoke hearts, halved

- 1 cup beef stock

- 1 red onion, sliced

- 1 cup tomato sauce

- ½ teaspoon rosemary, dried

- ½ teaspoon coriander, ground

- 1 teaspoon garlic powder

- A drizzle of olive oil

- A pinch of salt and black pepper

- 1 tablespoon chives, chopped

Directions:

1. Grease the slow cooker with the oil and mix the beef with the artichokes, stock and the other ingredients inside.

2. Toss, put the lid on and cook on High for 4 hours.

3. Divide the stew into bowls and serve.

Nutrition: calories 322, fat 5, fiber 4, carbs 12, protein 22

Pumpkin Chili

Preparation time: 10 minutes

Cooking time: 5 hours

Servings: 6

Ingredients:

- 1 cup pumpkin puree

- 30 ounces canned kidney beans, drained

- 30 ounces canned roasted tomatoes, chopped

- 2 cups water

- 1 cup red lentils, dried

- 1 cup yellow onion, chopped

- 1 jalapeno pepper, chopped

- 1 tablespoon chili powder

- 1 tablespoon cocoa powder

- ½ teaspoon cinnamon powder

- 2 teaspoons cumin, ground

- A pinch of cloves, ground

- Salt and black pepper to the taste

- 2 tomatoes, chopped

Directions:

1. In your Slow cooker, mix pumpkin puree with kidney beans, roasted tomatoes, water, lentils, onion, jalapeno, chili powder, cocoa, cinnamon, cumin, cloves, salt and pepper, stir, cover and cook on High for 5 hours.

2. Divide into bowls, top with chopped tomatoes and serve for lunch.

Nutrition: calories 266, fat 6, fiber 4, carbs 12, protein 4

Beef Soup

Preparation time: 10 minutes

Cooking time: 5 hours

Servings: 2

Ingredients:

- 1 pound beef stew meat, cubed

- 3 cups beef stock

- ½ cup tomatoes, cubed

- 1 red onion, chopped

- 1 green bell pepper, chopped

- 1 carrot, cubed

- A pinch of salt and black pepper

- ½ tablespoon oregano, dried

- ¼ teaspoon chili pepper

- 2 tablespoon tomato paste

- 1 jalapeno, chopped

- 1 tablespoon cilantro, chopped

Directions:

1. In your slow cooker, mix the beef with the stock, tomatoes and the other ingredients, toss, put the lid on and cook on Low for 5 hours.

2. Divide the soup into bowls and serve for lunch.

Nutrition: calories 391, fat 6, fiber 7, carbs 8, protein 27

Conclusion

Did you delight in trying these brand-new and scrumptious dishes? unfortunately we have come to the end of this vegan cookbook, I truly wish it has actually been to your liking. to boost your health and wellness we would love to recommend you to incorporate exercise and also a dynamic way of living along with follow these superb dishes, so as to emphasize the enhancements. we will certainly be back soon with other significantly intriguing vegan recipes, a big hug, see you soon.

CPSIA information can be obtained
at www.ICGtesting.com
Printed in the USA
BVHW061151280521
608377BV00001B/241